YOUNG PEOPLE LIVING WITH MENTAL ILLNESS

Learn How To Tell Your Parents

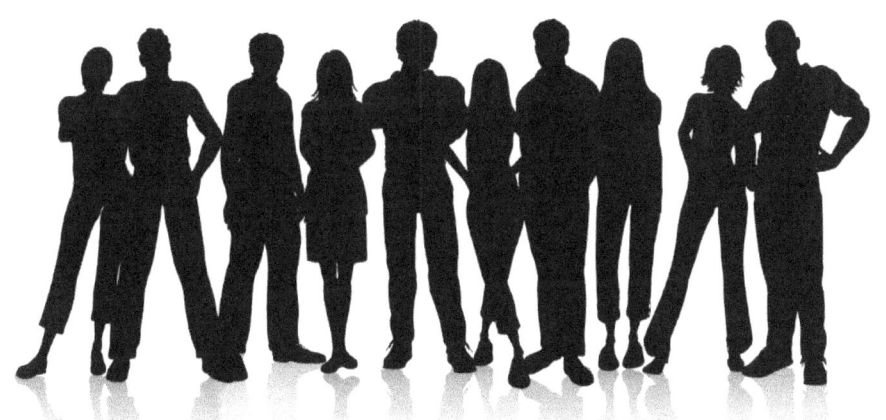

By Patricia A. Carlisle

Introduction

I want to thank you and congratulate you for choosing the book, *"YOUNG PEOPLE LIVING WITH MENTAL ILLNESS: Learn How to Tell Your Parents"*.

This book contains proven steps and strategies on how to tell your parents you have a mental illness.

Dealing with mental illness can be very difficult especially for young people. If you suspect you are one of them, you need to ask for help. The people, who are most willing to help you no matter what happens, are of course your parents.

Here comes the difficult part. Telling your parents can be a very hard task to accomplish. This is because they love you more than anything in the world, and it will affect them to know their son or daughter is going through a difficult time. All the same, you are not doing them any favor if you keep this a secret. Sooner or later they will find out because nobody knows you better. It is impossible to deal with the illness on your own, and you need their help.

Thanks again for choosing this book, I hope you enjoy it!

information is without contract or any type of guarantee assurance.

The trademarks that are used are without any consent, and the publication of the trademark is without permission or backing by the trademark owner. All trademarks and brands within this book are for clarifying purposes only and are the owned by the owners themselves, not affiliated with this document.

ABOUT THE AUTHOR
Patricia A. Carlisle, MSW, CBT

Patricia Carlisle- A Master Social Worker and a Cognitive Behavioral Therapist (CBT) gives out an expression of how important it is for an individual to take into consideration the concept of self-assessment to know what human, technical and conceptual skills they posses to perform or to achieve what they desire, or to deal with everyday life. However, every particular group of people has their own unique set of ideas, traditions and events including the frame of mind according to which people perform but there are many who faces problems and fail to maintain a healthy mind set affecting their behaviors and performance to those around them.

People like Patricia Carlisle are among those who have felt this urge of serving people and helping them out of their mental crisis towards a healthy life. She has experienced some close encounters in her personal life regarding mental health issues in her family and friends that has encouraged her to pursue this as her career.

Currently Patricia Carlisle is serving as a Certified On-Line Cognitive Behavioral Therapist with an extensive 15years of experience using Cognitive-Behavior Therapy Techniques. She envisions a world where everyone gets mental health treatment with no mental health stigma and to make it real she has already set up her own Holistic Measure Online Comprehensive Behavioral Healthcare Company after retiring from The Nord Center in The Partial Hospitalization Program (PHP) Dept for 5 years and Murtis H. Taylor Mental Health Center as a mental health counselor, psychological support technician and case manager for 10 years to emulsify her skills more professionally. Along with this, she has wrote down her passion as a clinician in 25 or more short books to help individuals and families get their life back, freeing them of the restraints of negative thinking, anxiety and depression by using different approaches. She is highly appreciated among her clients for her flexibility and professionalism of dealing with them graciously.

To reach her, make use of her direct website address: http://therapist2013.wix.com/e-therapy . As she is ready to inspire hope and contribute to health and well-being by providing the best online health care through comprehensive practice, education and research.

TABLE OF CONTENT

Chapter 1

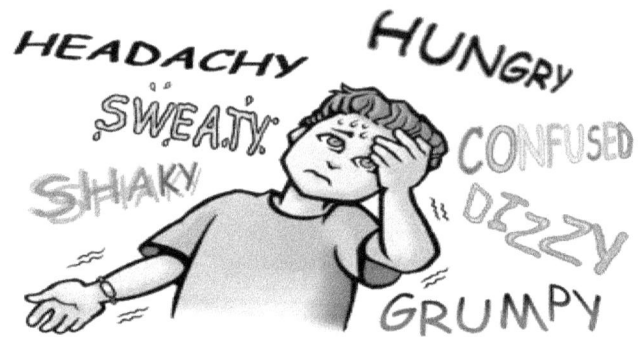

RECOGNIZE THE SYMPTOMS

Before telling your parents anything, first of all you need to know yourself. It is impossible to diagnose your own illness, and find out exactly what mental disease you have, but you can look out for some general symptoms. Try to figure out if your behavior changed in the last period of time.

A sudden change is an extra reason to suspect a mental illness. For example, before you used to be an outgoing person who loved to be surrounded by people. Now you can't stand to be in large groups. You prefer to be alone, and you might also have negative thoughts. If those thoughts are turning into suicidal thoughts, you need to tell your parents right away. Together you will go to a doctor and get the urgent help you need. Keeping these things inside can be very dangerous. Some mental illnesses can also cause hallucinations and delusions. You might also have recurring nightmares.

If you have any of these warning signs you will have to speak to your parents about it, and decide together the course of action. A deep sadness, also known as depression, is the most common symptom. You feel the need to spend time by yourself, and you hardly smile or have fun anymore. You can't find a good reason for your sadness, and this might scare you.

While before you used to be very active, and you loved to go out with your friends, now they are telling you how much you've changed. The only thing you want to do is lock yourself in your room and sleep.

Being tired all the time can also be a worrying sign. Some young people can sleep many hours a day, or they can have problems falling asleep. A change in the way you eat can also occur. For example, you can start eating a lot more or less than before. You can also feel that you can't cope with the daily routine like going to school, cleaning, doing homework or other chores. Do not confuse this with laziness. Being lazy means you can do all those things, but you simply don't want to do it. When you are suffering with a mental illness you might find it impossible to do these simple tasks. If that is the case, and your parents are mad at you, the only solution is to tell them exactly how you feel. Make them understand that you would like to do your chores, but you are unable to. Explain to them everything that you feel, and ask for their help. Make sure you give them as many details as possible. If at first they don't understand, try not to get disappointed. Keep on insisting until you make things clear.

It is very possible that they will not understand. In this case, do not get mad at them or disappointed. They still love you very much, but they are not doctors. It is difficult for people without any knowledge about mental illness to understand. They might need some time to take in the information too. Be patient because they are your parents, and in the end they will not let you down.

Another symptom is being short tempered. If you feel you are easily getting angry, and you don't find an explanation for it, a mental illness could be the cause. One of the most common mental illnesses is the Bipolar disorder. The most common signs for this disease are the extreme mood swings. A person might be in a great mood in one second only to change completely in the next second. This is only one example of a mental illness. The worse mistake you can do is to start guessing the name of your illness. This is the doctor's job. Yours is just to find out if you have any worrying signs, and to communicate them to your parents. A mental illness discovered in time can be easier to keep under control. This means you can start treatment right away, and spare yourself and your parents from suffering.

Anxiety is another big symptom that is present with various mental illnesses. This anxiety or fear makes its appearance especially when you are in public spaces. In this case it is better to avoid big crowds. Isolating yourself from all people is not beneficial, but if you feel that you can't handle this yet this is okay. The two people you should never avoid are your mother and father. No matter how you feel, you need them by your side. Anxiety can manifest as a panic attack, or a sensation of fear. It is also possible to have difficulty breathing, and some people can even pass out during an anxiety attack. You will not have any logical explanation for this fear. The good news is that you can take a treatment to relief anxiety symptoms. The treatment is in the form of pills or coping skills. Any treatment you take needs to be prescribed by a doctor.

Chapter 2

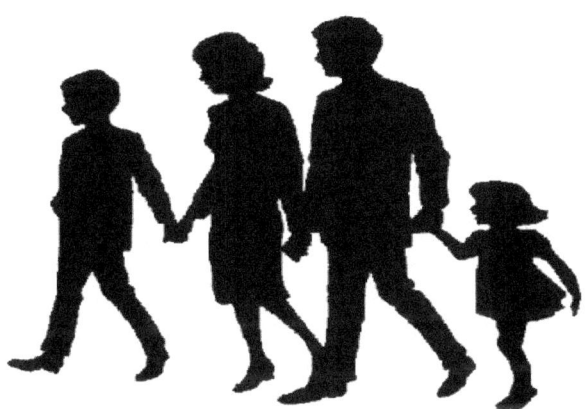

COMMUNICATE WITH YOUR PARENTS

For young people, especially teenagers, it can be difficult to maintain good communication with their parents. The age gap, and the difference in mentality between generations can make it difficult to talk about anything. However, you should always make an effort especially when it comes to discussing your health. No matter how mad they drive you, keep in mind there is no one else on this earth that cares about you more than they do.

If you have warning signs that make you believe you might be suffering of a mental illness, ask your parents to sit down, and listen to what you have to say. Start by explaining to them how you are feeling. Describe in detail the symptoms, and dark thoughts you are having. Try to keep calm when you are talking to them. If the discussion escalates into a new fight, you will not be able to make them understand that you need help. Be patient with them. There is nothing they wouldn't do for you, but they are not mind readers. Communicate your problems to them is your job.

Do not spare any detail. Before you talk to them, make a list with all your thoughts and feelings. This way, if the discussion gets too emotional, you will not miss any important information. You need to realize that what you are about to tell them will make them feel sad. Tears are inevitable, and you need to be okay with that. They will only be sad because they don't want you to suffer. This does not mean you did anything to disappoint them. A mental illness, like any other type of illness, is out of your control, and you shouldn't blame yourself.

Many young people with mental illnesses might feel too embarrassed to admit this to anyone. However, your parents are not just anyone. It is okay if you don't want to discuss this with anyone else. People can be very judgmental. With your father and mother you are safe. Open up to them and share your fears. Knowing that you don't have to go through this alone can make you feel much better.

You might even have a pleasant surprise to hear that some of the things you are experiencing are perfectly normal. However, if you feel something is not right, be firm on the subject, and find a solution together. The best thing you can do together is to go see a doctor. At the appointment, make sure your parents are in the room so they can better understand your condition. Remember that while they are older and wiser than you are, they are still not medical professionals. Hearing explanations from a doctor can help them understand better. A doctor can also give them the tools they need to help you.

Chapter 3

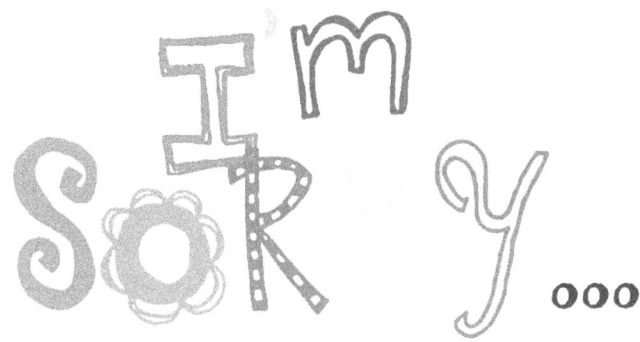

APOLOGIZE AHEAD OF TIME FOR YOUR BEHAVIOR

Being short tempered or angry can be one of the many symptoms of your mental illness. Whenever you are feeling calm that is the time to talk to your parents about it. Explain to them how you feel whenever you cannot control you anger.

Tell them that you are very sorry for this, and that you don't want to hurt them. This way, next time it happens they will understand you better, and they will have more patience with you.

A doctor can teach you how to cope with your feelings of anger and despair. After you take your treatment (medication), and you go to therapy, you will have the possibility to control yourself just like a healthy person. Therefore, keep in mind that how you feel today can change for the better tomorrow. Everything is only temporary, and you are strong enough to overcome the illness. There is no need for despair, or to give up.

There are some simple coping exercises you can do by yourself at home before you even get help from a doctor. For example, you can count slowly to ten. Do this whenever you feel that you are losing your patience, and starting to get angry. If this doesn't work, combine the counting with slow breathing. Breathe in and out and count while you do it. This way you will be focusing on what your body is doing, and your mind will calm down before you know it. Going in another room or another place is also beneficial. This way you are getting away from the thing or person that got you angry in the first place.

If you feel that you can control your anger, do it. It is a lot easier to go out of control and react. However, you need to remember that you are hurting yourself, and the people you love. Getting in control can be more difficult for you than it is for a healthy person, but you need to keep fighting. Do not use the mental illness as an excuse for your behavior. You get in control by getting to know yourself better. For example, pay attention to the things that make you angry. Those are call triggers. If you can avoid these, you are already one step ahead.

Create a calm environment for yourself. Avoid anything that has to do with violence including movies and video games. If you have a friend in your life that always manages to push your buttons, try to avoid him or her for the time you are under treatment. The only people you cannot hide from are your parents. This is why it is essential for them to understand what you are going through.

Chapter 4

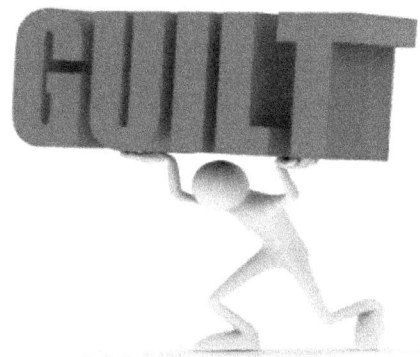

DO NOT FEEL GUILTY

When you are suffering from mental illness, you can say or do things you don't really mean. This can end up hurting people around you. When these people are your own parents, the pain is even greater. It is very easy to feel guilty. However, you need to remember that the illness is taking over your mind. That was not really you, and your parents understand this. Feelings of guilt and shame will only delay the process of healing. Your only goal should be to find the right course of treatment, and get back to being yourself soon. Do not dwell on the past. Whatever you said or did yesterday should stay in the past.

Set up small milestones and goals for yourself. For example, you can keep a notebook to write down the way you feel every day. If you started a treatment for your illness, and you notice that a day went by and you felt great, celebrate it. That is your little victory, and days like that will help you get better. If you have a bad day, remember the good times, and try to do better in the future. Thinking about how you behaved badly will not help. It is always better to focus your attention on the positive things. The bad days are a reaction of the illness, and you are not responsible for them. Your only duty is to get better, and you can do it. With the support of your parents there isn't anything you can't do.

If you had some moments of anger when you raised the tone of your voice to your parents, wait until you calm down before you talk to them. When you feel at peace again, try to explain to them what you felt during those moments when you lost your temper. Talking about things can help you and your parents move past them. If this repeats in the near future, your parents will have a better understanding about your illness. They will know how to handle your anger attacks. Maybe they can even help you avoid them altogether.

Chapter 5

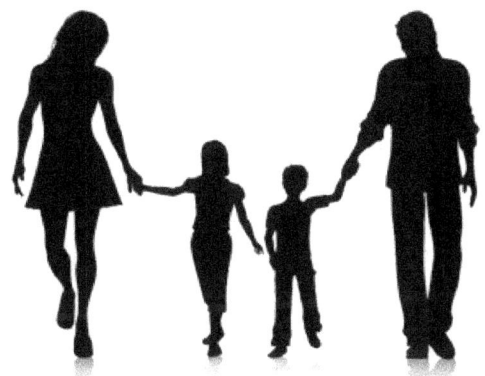

GO TOGETHER TO A DOCTOR

Once you had the conversation about your symptoms, it is time to look for help from a person who knows more about mental illness. This person of course, is a doctor. Your parents might not be able to join you at every appointment, but the first one is very important. They will have the chance to ask the doctor anything they want. Because they are older, that don't mean they know everything. Most of the time they may be as scared and confused as you are. A better understanding over the illness can help you and your parents cope with it better. Meet with more than one doctor. This will allow you to choose the one you are most at ease with. The relationship you form with a therapist can be on a very personal level. He or she will be hearing your deepest thoughts and feelings. You might learn new things about yourself too. Because of this you should make sure that you are comfortable with the doctor you choose.

After a few sessions, if you feel your parents still need help understand and helping you, invite them to assist you to some more of your doctor's appointments. They can go to talk to the doctor on their own as well. There are also support groups for families. Encourage them to join one of those groups too. It can be very difficult to understand something you are not experiencing yourself. This doesn't mean your illness doesn't affect them too. On some level, parents are hurting even more whenever their children are ill.

There is no need for them to be present to all the therapy sessions you have. Sometimes you might feel the need to speak your mind without them hearing. That is okay. Everybody needs a little privacy from time to time. After each session, tell your parents everything you learned. A therapist will teach you how to cope with the symptoms and this is information your parents need to have too.

Chapter 6

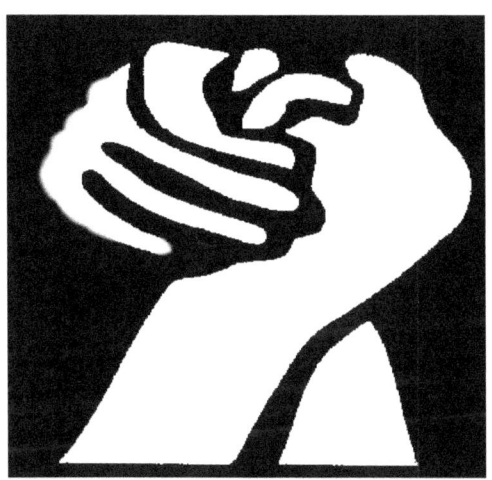

RESEARCH MENTAL ILLNESS TOGETHER

If you get a diagnosis from a doctor, the next step is to learn as many things as possible about that specific mental illness. If you don't understand it, it can be difficult to treat it. Do this together with your parents. Don't leave them out of it because it affects them as much as it affects you. There are plenty books you can get to help you learn about the illness and its symptoms. Your doctor will also give you material to read.

Take your time to study everything, and don't hesitate to ask questions. Some medical terms can be difficult to understand.

You can also find the information you need online. Search for forums where you can chat with other people suffering of the same illness or with their families. You can discover their experiences and they might have some good coping tips for you. However, it is important to not believe everything you read on forums. Each person is unique and while some symptoms are the same for you too, others can be different. You should consider the online forums as support groups. If you need real information you will need to ask a doctor.

Ask your doctor if there are any real support groups you can join together with your parents. Talking to friends can be beneficial too but they can never really understand. Your parents can talk to other parents who have more experience with that specific mental illness. You will have the opportunity to communicate with other young people going through the same thing as you are. You will not only get valuable tips, but talking to someone who understands your illness can make you feel better. An illness can make you feel very lonely. Knowing that others are in the same situation will give you the strength you need to fight.

Conclusion

Thank you again for choosing this book!

I hope this book was able to help you to find the courage to discuss your mental health with your parents.

Your mental illness can affect the entire family and especially your parents. It takes a lot of courage to tell them about your mental illness but it is something you really need to do. If your behavior changed recently they already suspect that something is wrong with you. Do not let them guess because this can make them worry even more. With their help you can find the courage to move past it and get better. Living with a mental illness can be very scary.

Luckily, your mom and dad are there for you. All you need to do is reach out to them. They will support you whenever you feel like you cannot go on.

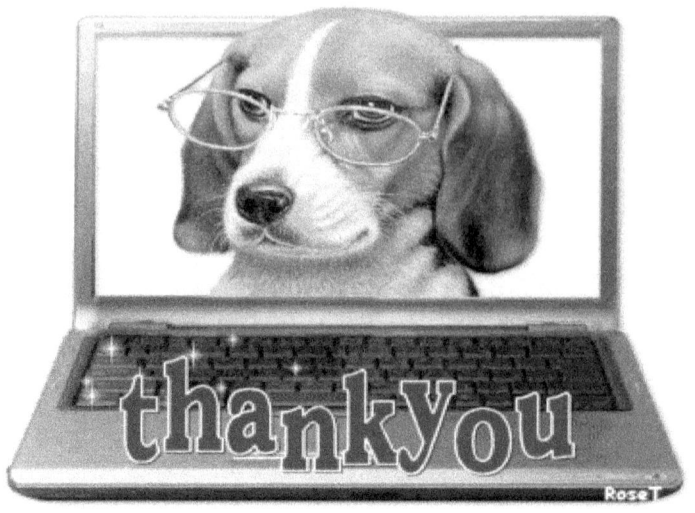

Finally, if you enjoyed this book, would you be kind enough to leave a review for this book on Amazon.com. It'd be greatly appreciated!

Thank you and good luck!

Preview Of 'THE DEPRESSION CURE: How to overcome depression and Become Depression Free'

Chapter 1: MOOD DISORDER
Tackling depression head-on the right way

Recovery begins when we overcome depression and become totally depression free. Treatment for depression starts when one recognizes the symptoms and began to seek help. To find a Depression cure it requires patience from both the individual and the physician. Depression is not like normal sadness and happiness if you are experiencing feelings of despair, or hopelessness. Most people do not realize they are depressed and let this illness go unnoticed.

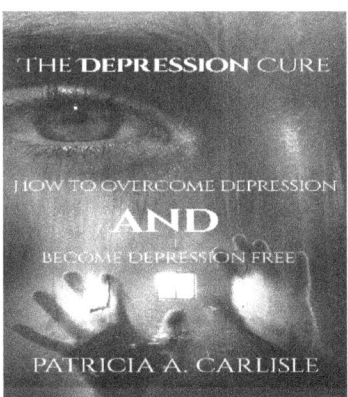

THE DEPRESSION CURE: How to overcome depression and become depression free,

Check Out My Other Books

Below you'll find some of my other popular books that are popular on Amazon and Kindle as well. Alternatively, you can visit my author page on Amazon to see other work done by me. (https://amazon.com/author/patriciacarlisle)

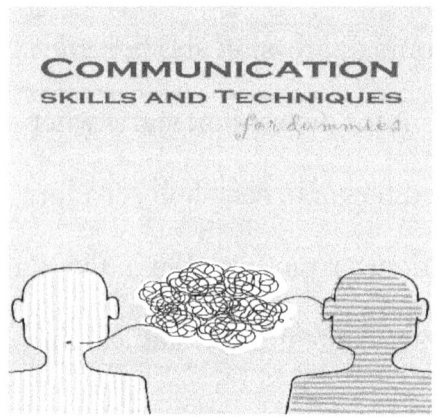

COMMUNICATION SKILLS AND TECHNIQUES FOR DUMMIES.

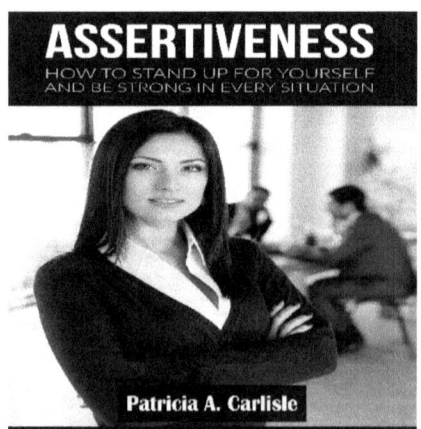

ASSERTIVENESS: How to stand up for yourself and be strong in every situation.

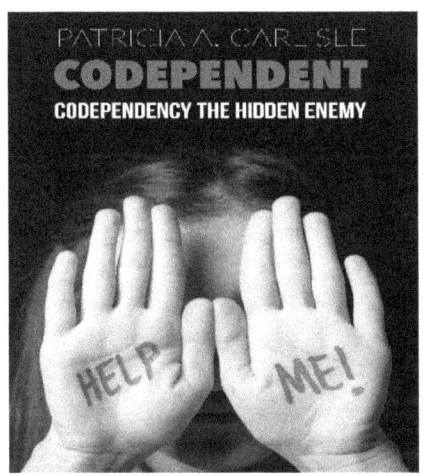

Codependent: Codependency the Hidden Enemy.

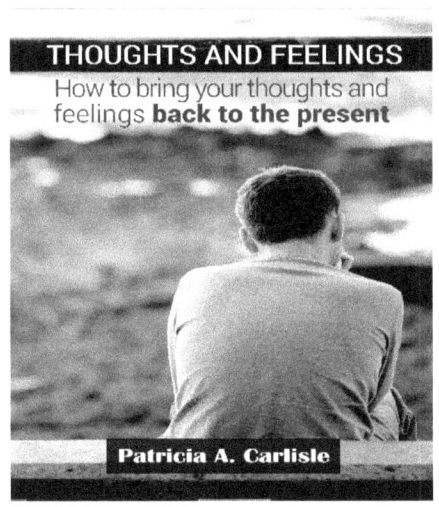

THOUGHTS-FEELINGS: How to bring your thoughts and feelings back to the present.

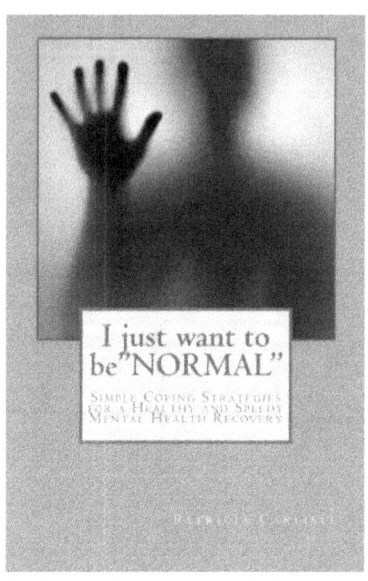

I just want to be "NORMAL" Simple Coping Strategies for a Healthy and Speedy Mental Health Recovery.

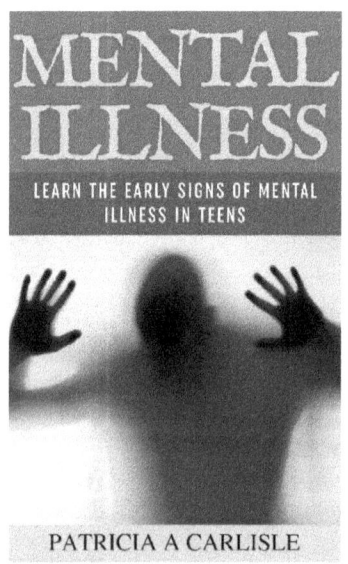

MENTAL Illness: LEARN THE EARLY SIGNS OF MENTAL ILLNESS IN TEENS.

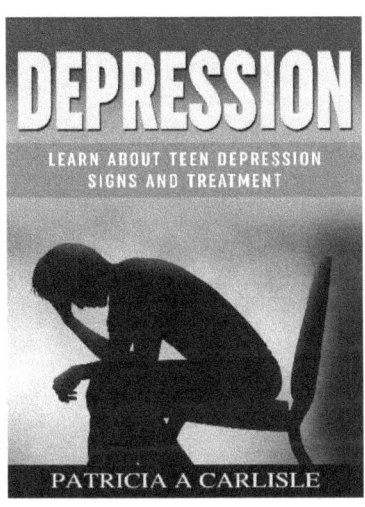

DEPRESSION: LEARN ABOUT TEEN DEPRESSION SIGNS AND TREATMENT.

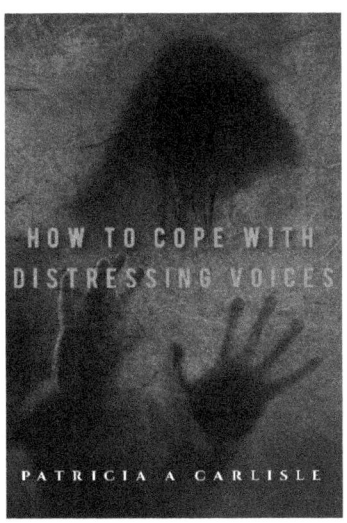

HOW TO COPE WITH DISTRESSING VOICES.

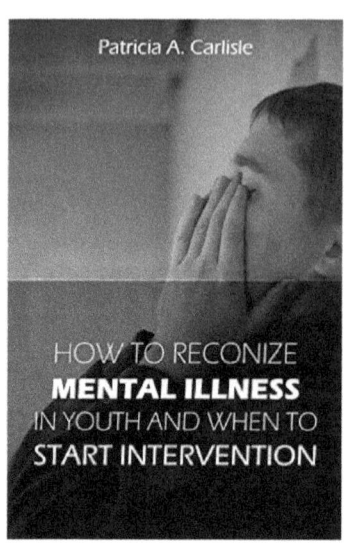

MENTAL ILLNESS: HOW TO RECOGNIZE MENTAL
ILLNESS IN YOUTH AND WHEN TO START
INTERVENTION.

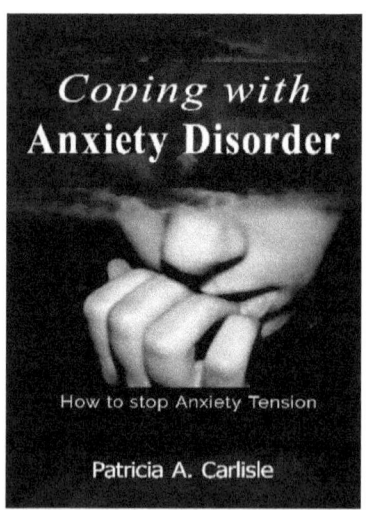

COPING WITH ANXIETY DISORDER: HOW TO
STOP ANXIETY TENSION.

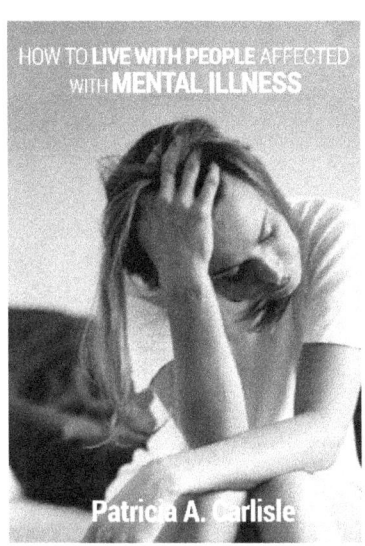

HOW TO LIVE WITH PEOPLE AFFECTED WITH MENTAL ILLNESS.

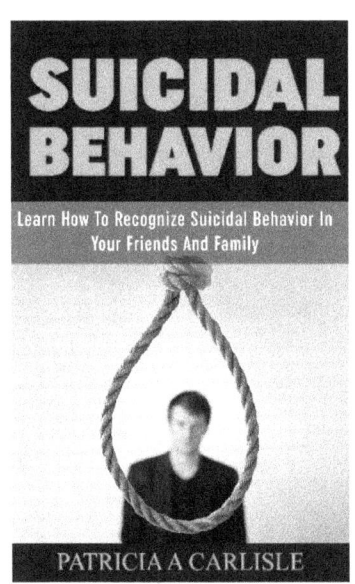

SUICIDAL BEHAVIOR: LEARN HOW TO RECOGNIZE SUICISAL BEHAVIOR IN YOUR FRIENDS AND FAMILY.

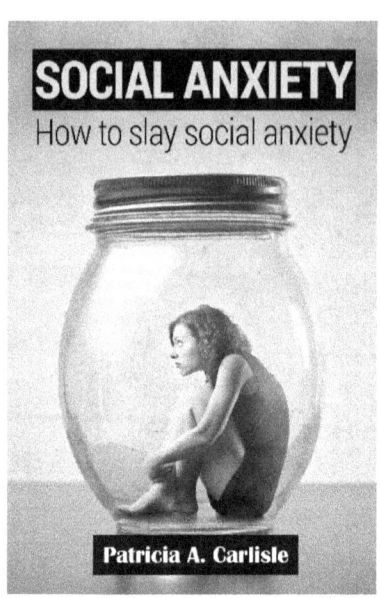

SOCIAL ANXIETY: HOW TO SLAY SOCIAL ANXIETY.

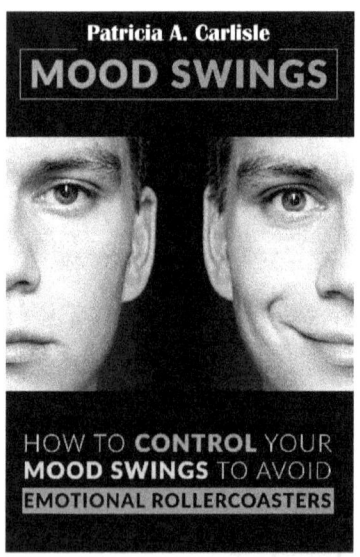

MOOD SWINGS: HOW TO CONTROL YOUR MOOD SWINGS TO AVOID EMOTIONAL ROLLERCOASTER'S.

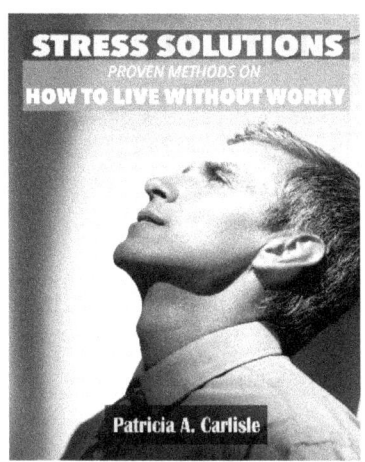

**STRESS SOLUTONS: PROVEN METHODS ON HOW
TO LIVE WITHOUT WORRY.**

BONUS: SUBSCRIBE TO THE FREE BOOK

Beginners Guide to Yoga & Meditation

"Stressed out? Do You Feel Like The World Is Crashing Down Around You? Want To Take A Vacation That Will Relax Your Mind, Body And Spirit? Well this Easy To Read Step By Step

E-Book Makes It All Possible!"

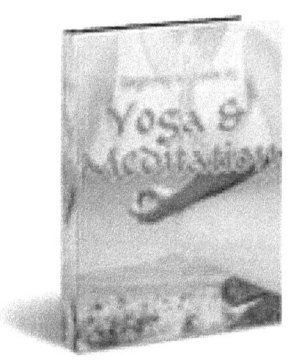

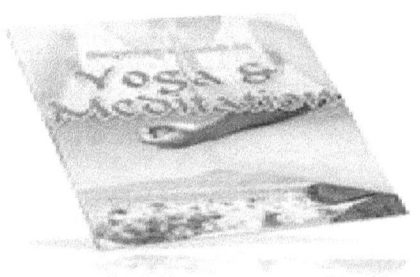

Instructions on how to join our mailing list, and receive a free copy of "Yoga and Meditation" can be found in any of my Kindle eBooks.

NOTES

NOTES

NOTES

NOTES

NOTES

NOTES

NOTES

NOTES

www.ingramcontent.com/pod-product-compliance
Lightning Source LLC
Chambersburg PA
CBHW071019180526
45168CB00003B/1491